Redefining Health: A Guide To Achieve Hormone Balance And Reclaim Vitality Naturally

Elizabeth J. Drumm

Acknowledgements

Writing "Redefining Health: A Guide to Achieve Hormone Balance and Reclaim Vitality Naturally" has been a transformative journey, one that would not have been possible without the guidance, support, and inspiration from many extraordinary individuals.

First and foremost, I would like to express my deepest gratitude to the giants in the field of health, fitness, and natural medicine whose groundbreaking work has profoundly influenced my own. Dr. Christiane Northrup, your pioneering insights into women's health and hormones have been a beacon of wisdom. Dr. Mark Hyman, your dedication to functional medicine and holistic health has reshaped the way we approach wellness. Dr. Sara Gottfried, your expertise in hormone balancing has provided invaluable knowledge and inspiration. Dr. Joseph Mercola, your relentless pursuit of natural health solutions has been a constant source of motivation.

To my family, words cannot adequately express my appreciation for your unwavering support and encouragement throughout this journey. To my loving spouse, thank you for your patience, understanding, and belief in me, even during the late nights and early mornings spent writing. To my children, your enthusiasm and curiosity have been a constant source of joy and motivation. And to my parents, your lifelong dedication to health and wellness instilled in me the values that have guided this work.

A special thanks to my friends and colleagues who provided invaluable feedback and encouragement. Your insights and suggestions have helped shape this book into what it is today.

Lastly, to my readers, thank you for your trust and interest in this journey towards achieving hormone balance and natural vitality. It is my hope that this book will empower you to take

charge of your health and live your most vibrant life.
With heartfelt gratitude,
Elizabeth J. Drumm

Introduction

In this modern time, few subjects are as captivating and vital as understanding the intricate dance of hormones within our bodies. Imagine a symphony where each instrument plays a crucial role in harmony, influencing everything from our mood and energy levels to our metabolism and reproductive health. This book is your backstage pass to unraveling the mysteries of hormone balance—a journey that promises empowerment, vitality, and a deeper connection with your body's inner workings.

Picture this: You wake up feeling refreshed, with your mind clear and your body vibrant with energy. Throughout the day, you navigate tasks effortlessly, fueled by a steady stream of focus and productivity. Your mood is stable, your skin glows with vitality, and you feel in tune with your emotions. This is the promise of hormone balance—a state where your body's chemical messengers work in perfect synchrony, supporting optimal health and well-being.

Yet, for many, this ideal feels elusive. The reality is often marked by fatigue that refuses to lift, mood swings that derail even the best-laid plans, and a sense of disconnect from one's own body. Hormone imbalance manifests in myriad ways—irregular menstrual cycles, stubborn weight gain, sleep disturbances, and even more serious conditions like infertility or thyroid disorders. It's a journey through peaks and valleys, where understanding becomes the compass guiding us towards restoration and vitality.

This book is not just a collection of facts and figures but a roadmap—a comprehensive guide crafted to empower you on your quest for hormone balance. Whether you're navigating the tumultuous seas of puberty, striving for fertility, weathering the storm of menopause, or simply seeking to optimize your health, the principles within these pages will illuminate your path.

Here, we delve deep into the intricate web of hormones, exploring their roles and interactions within the body. From estrogen and progesterone to insulin, cortisol, and thyroid hormones, each plays a crucial part in regulating various bodily functions. Understanding these roles empowers you to make informed choices—whether in nutrition, lifestyle, or medical interventions—that support hormone balance and overall well-being.

But this book is more than a scientific exploration; it's a testament to the resilience of the human body and spirit. It's about reclaiming control over your health and embracing a holistic approach that nurtures not just physical vitality but also mental clarity and emotional equilibrium. It invites you to cultivate a deeper relationship with your body—to listen to its whispers and respond with kindness and wisdom.

Throughout these pages, you'll discover practical strategies backed by the latest research and clinical insights. From hormone-balancing diet plans and targeted supplements to stress management techniques and mindful practices, each recommendation is designed to be actionable and transformative. You'll learn how small, intentional changes in lifestyle can yield profound results in restoring hormone balance and reclaiming your vitality.

Moreover, this book addresses the interconnectedness of hormone balance with other aspects of health—such as gut health, inflammation, and the impact of environmental toxins. It sheds light on how these factors influence hormonal harmony and provides strategies to mitigate their effects, ensuring a comprehensive approach to wellness.

Imagine stepping into a world where hormone balance isn't just a concept but a lived reality—a state where you feel empowered, energized, and in sync with your body's natural rhythms. This book is your guide to making that vision a reality. It's a toolkit filled with knowledge, insights, and practical advice to support you on every step of your journey towards hormone balance and vibrant health.

As you embark on this transformative journey, remember: you hold the power to reshape your health and well-being. By embracing the principles outlined in these pages and taking proactive steps towards nurturing your hormones, you're not just reclaiming vitality—you're rewriting the narrative of your health journey. Let this book be your companion, your mentor, and your inspiration as you embark on this empowering quest towards optimal hormone balance and a life lived in full harmony with your body.

Chapter 1

Hormones are intricate chemical messengers that orchestrate and regulate a wide range of physiological processes in the human body. They are produced by specific glands and tissues located throughout the body, which together form the endocrine system. This system works in tandem with the neurological system to provide exact coordination and control over physiological functions and behaviors.

Hormones' principal role is to transfer signals from one portion of the body to another. Endocrine glands such as the pituitary gland, thyroid gland, adrenal glands, pancreas, ovaries, and testes release them directly into the bloodstream, as do some tissues such as the kidneys, liver, and adipose tissue. Hormones then circulate throughout the body, binding to receptor molecules on target cells or organs.

Hormones, once linked to their receptors, cause a cascade of metabolic processes within target cells, resulting in specific physiological responses. These reactions might vary from changing gene expression and protein synthesis to regulating cell metabolism and influencing growth and development.

Hormones have a wide range of impacts, influencing almost every area of human health and well-being. Hormones, for example, govern metabolism by directing how foods are used and energy is stored. They also play an important role in regulating mood, emotions, and behavior, impacting processes like stress response, sleep habits, and cognition.

Furthermore, hormones play an important role in reproductive and sexual development. In males, the testes generate testosterone, which promotes the development of secondary sexual characteristics and regulates sperm production. In females, the ovaries produce estrogen and progesterone, which regulate menstrual cycles, support pregnancy, and help develop secondary sexual characteristics.

Hormonal balance and appropriate function are critical for sustaining homeostasis, or internal balance, in the body. Hormone imbalances, whether caused by aging, stress, disease, or environmental factors, can result in a variety of health problems. Diabetes, thyroid diseases, infertility, and mood disorders are all common conditions linked to hormonal imbalance.

In conclusion, hormones are important chemical messengers that act as the body's internal communication system, orchestrating and coordinating vital physiological processes. Their delicate regulation and balance are critical to overall health and well-being, emphasizing the need for understanding and maintaining hormonal health to ensure optimal physical functioning.

Understanding your body's hormones and functions.

Understanding your body's hormones and their actions is critical for understanding how various physiological processes are controlled and maintained. Hormones are chemical messengers produced by specialized glands and tissues throughout the body, forming the endocrine system. They serve an important role in coordinating and managing a wide range of body functions, including metabolism, growth, mood, and reproductive processes.

1. Endocrine Glands and Hormone Production: The pituitary, thyroid, adrenal, pancreatic, ovarian, and testicular glands are responsible for hormone production. In addition, several organs, such as the kidneys, liver, and adipose tissue, create hormones.

Each gland produces hormones that perform various tasks in the body.

2. Mode of Action: Hormones are released into the bloodstream and delivered to specific cells or organs throughout the body. They attach to specific receptors on target cells' surfaces or within the cell. This binding causes biochemical events inside the cells, resulting in a variety of physiological responses.

3. Key Hormones and Their Functions:

- Insulin: The pancreas produces insulin, which regulates blood sugar levels by promoting glucose uptake into cells for energy production.

- Thyroid Hormones: The thyroid gland secretes these hormones, which govern metabolism, growth, and development.

- Adrenal Hormones (Cortisol and Adrenaline): Cortisol, produced by the adrenal glands, aids in the regulation of stress and metabolism, whereas adrenaline activates the "fight or flight" response.

- Sex Hormones (Estrogen, Progesterone, and Testosterone): The ovaries predominantly generate estrogen and progesterone, which regulate menstrual periods and reproductive activities in females. In males, testosterone is primarily produced by the testes and stimulates the development of male secondary sexual traits while also regulating sperm production.

4. Regulation and Feedback Mechanisms: The brain system and endocrine glands work together to closely regulate hormone levels. Negative feedback loops keep hormone levels within a small range, allowing the body to maintain homeostasis, or internal balance.

5. Imbalances in hormone synthesis or signaling might cause health concerns. Hypothyroidism (low thyroid hormone levels) can induce weariness, weight gain, and cold sensitivity, whereas hyperthyroidism (excess thyroid

hormone) can result in weight loss, rapid heartbeat, and heat intolerance.

Diabetes, infertility, mental problems, and osteoporosis are all illnesses that can be caused by hormonal abnormalities.

6. Factors Influencing Hormonal Health: Age, genetics, stress, nutrition, exercise, medications, and environmental exposure can all impact hormonal balance. Understanding these impacts can help people make more educated lifestyle decisions that promote hormonal health.

Hormones are required to sustain the body's overall health and function. Understanding their functions and interactions enables people to take proactive steps to promote hormonal balance through lifestyle changes, medical changes and appropriate healthcare interventions.

Women hormones and weight

Women's hormones regulate metabolism, hunger, and fat storage, all of which influence body weight and composition.

Several essential hormones, principally produced by the ovaries, adrenal glands, and other organs, help to regulate these processes.

1. Estrogen is the main female hormone that regulates the menstrual cycle, reproductive activities, and other physiological processes. It regulates fat distribution and metabolism. Prior to menopause, estrogen promotes fat deposition in places such as the hips and thighs, contributing to the typical female body shape. However, estrogen levels change throughout the menstrual cycle, and these variations can have various effects on hunger and energy expenditure, depending on the phase.

2. Progesterone works with estrogen to control the menstrual cycle and promote pregnancy. It also influences metabolism, which may affect weight gain or loss. Progesterone levels rise during pregnancy and the second half of the menstrual cycle, influencing hunger and

potentially increasing calorie consumption. In some women, progesterone causes increased water retention and bloating, which may have a brief impact on weight.

3. Insulin: Although not a female hormone, insulin is vital for metabolism and weight regulation. It is produced by the pancreas and helps to regulate blood sugar levels. Insulin levels are elevated in situations such as insulin resistance, which is more common in women with polycystic ovarian syndrome (PCOS). This might cause weight gain, especially around the abdomen.

4. Cortisol: The adrenal glands create cortisol in response to stress, which regulates metabolism and fat storage. Chronic stress can raise cortisol levels, increase hunger, particularly for high-calorie foods, and promote fat storage, especially around the abdomen. High cortisol levels may contribute to weight gain in some

women.

5. Thyroid Hormones: Thyroid hormones, including thyroxine (T4) and triiodothyronine (T3), regulate metabolism and energy consumption. Thyroid problems, such as hypothyroidism (underactive thyroid) or hyperthyroidism (overactive thyroid), can impact metabolism and cause weight changes. Hypothyroidism, which is more frequent in women, slows metabolism and contributes to weight gain, whereas hyperthyroidism promotes weight loss.

6. Leptin and Ghrelin: These hormones help regulate hunger and satiety. Fat cells create leptin, which signals to the brain that you are full and can lower hunger. The stomach produces ghrelin, which stimulates appetite. Imbalances in these hormones might impair appetite control, perhaps resulting in weight gain or trouble reducing weight.

7. Menopause: At roughly age

50, estrogen and progesterone levels decrease considerably. This hormonal shift can alter body composition, resulting in increased belly fat and decreased lean muscle mass. These changes can lead to weight gain and a shift in fat distribution, which increases the risk of metabolic illnesses like insulin resistance and cardiovascular disease.

In conclusion, women's hormones have complex functions in regulating metabolism, hunger, fat accumulation, and body weight. Hormonal fluctuations during the menstrual cycle, pregnancy, and menopause can have varying effects on these systems at different periods of life. Understanding how hormones interact with lifestyle factors like nutrition, exercise, stress management, and sleep can help women manage their weight more successfully and promote overall hormonal health.

Iodine plays an important role in hormonal health,

particularly   for   women.

Iodine is a trace mineral that the body requires to produce thyroid hormones, which are necessary for proper growth and development. The thyroid gland in the neck contains approximately 70 to 80% of your body's iodine. The remainder is spread throughout the body, primarily in the ovaries, muscles, and blood. If your body does not have enough iodine, you may get hypothyroidism (low thyroid hormone levels). Symptoms include sluggishness or weariness, weight gain, dry skin, and temperature sensitivity. Deficiency affects more women than men, and it is more prevalent in pregnant women and older children. Hypothyroidism in newborns and children can impact both their physical and mental growth. Premature infants are more sensitive to iodine shortages because they are prematurely separated from their mother's iodine supply.

The hallmark symptom of iodine deficiency is an enlarged thyroid gland. Some people with hypothyroidism develop an unusually large thyroid, known as a goiter. Iodine deficiency is now uncommon in the United States and other industrialized countries due to the addition of iodine to table salt. Crops in affluent countries are often grown in iodine-rich soil therefore, food contains more iodine. More than 1 billion individuals in developing nations, where soil is frequently low in iodine, may be at risk of iodine deficiency.

Uses: Most people acquire enough iodine. Because of the complex way iodine affects the thyroid, you should not take iodine supplements unless your doctor advises you to. Iodine can be used to treat the following conditions:

Oral mucositis (oral irritation). Some data suggests that an iodine mouth rinse may alleviate symptoms of mucositis in the mouth caused by chemotherapy or radiation therapy.

Fibrocystic breast alterations. Some data suggests that iodine may be beneficial in treating fibrocystic breast disease. Women with fibrocystic breast disease have breast soreness, especially before their periods. A review of clinical research discovered that iodine replacement therapy (especially for patients with low iodine levels) may alleviate the soreness associated with fibrocystic breast tissue. The women who took iodine reported very few negative effects.

Vaginitis
Some women with chronic vaginal complaints utilize over-the-counter (OTC) iodine douches to relieve vaginal irritation, itching, and discharge. Povidone-iodine provides the benefits of iodine without the stinging and staining risks.

Wounds
Iodine is commonly used to disinfect the skin and clean wounds. Doctors routinely use iodine-based ointments on burns to reduce the risk of infection.

Radiation Exposure
Potassium iodine can be administered after radiation exposure to minimize radioactive iodine accumulation in the thyroid. This action lessens the chance of thyroid cancer caused by radiation exposure, but it does not protect against other radiation-related problems.

Prevention of Goiter
Iodine shortages can cause thyroid enlargement, often known as goiter. However, too much iodine can cause goiter. In developed countries, goiters caused by iodine deficiency are rare.

Dietary Resources
Iodized salt is the primary source of iodine in the diet. Shellfish, white deep-water fish, and brown seaweed kelp are all excellent providers of iodine because they absorb it from the water. Garlic, lima beans, sesame seeds, soybeans, spinach, Swiss chard, summer squash, and turnip greens are also rich in iodine. Bakeries may also add iodine to

dough as a stabilizing agent, providing bread with an additional source of iodine.

Available Forms

Sodium iodide (iodine) is available as a multivitamin/mineral supplement or as a topical wound therapy. Iodine is also found in seaweed-based nutritional supplements like kelp and bladderwrack.

How to Take It

The National Institute of Medicine Adequate Intake (AI) levels are as below:

Infants

Infants, ages 0 to 6 months: 110 mcg (micrograms) per day

Infants, ages 7 months to 1 year: 130 mcg per day

RDA (Recommended Dietary Amounts) have been established for children and adults.

Children

Children, ages 1 to 8 years: 90 mcg per day

Children, ages 9 to 13 years: 120 mcg per day

Children, ages 14 to 18 years: 150 mcg per day

Adult

Ages 18 years and up: 150 mcg per day

Pregnant females: 220 mcg per day

Breastfeeding women: 290 mcg per day

The following are Tolerable Uptake Intake Levels (UL), the highest level of daily intake that is not likely to result in side effects:

Children, 1 to 3 years: 200 mcg per day

Children, 4 to 8 years: 300 mcg per day

Children, 9 to 13 years: 600 mcg per day

From 14 to 18 years (including pregnant and breastfeeding women): 900 mcg day

For adults, older than 19 (including pregnant and breastfeeding women): 1,100 mcg per day

Wounds or burns: Follow your doctor's instructions. Iodine is applied topically to the skin to prevent and treat infections from wounds and burns.

Side effects:

When taken orally, iodine is likely safe for most people in quantities of less than 1100 mcg per day. Iodine taken in large doses or for an extended period of time may be harmful. Adults should avoid taking greater doses over an extended period of time unless they are under medical care. A higher intake may increase the chance of adverse effects, such as thyroid issues. Larger doses of iodine can cause a metallic taste, pain in the teeth and gums, burning in the mouth and throat, stomach discomfort, and a variety of other side effects.

When used in properly diluted formulations on the skin, iodine is likely safe for the majority of people. A 2% iodine solution is an FDA-approved prescription medication.

Special Precautions and Warnings:
Pregnancy and breastfeeding: Iodine is likely safe when taken orally at specified levels or applied to the skin using an approved product (2% solution). Above 18, do not take more than 1100 mcg of iodine per day; 14–18, do not take more than 900.

High quantities of iodine taken orally may be hazardous. Increased consumption may cause the baby to develop thyroid disorders.

Thyroid diseases: Prolonged or high doses of iodine may exacerbate some thyroid disorders, such as hypothyroidism, an enlarged thyroid gland (goiter), or a thyroid tumor. Furthermore, those with autoimmune thyroid illnesses may be particularly vulnerable to the negative effects of iodine.

Chapter 2

Understanding Hormone Imbalance

Hormone imbalance occurs when there are abnormalities in the body's normal production, release, or action of hormones, resulting in dysregulation of several physiological systems.

Hormones are vital chemical messengers that coordinate and control a wide range of functions, including metabolism, growth, mood, and reproduction. Their balance is critical to preserving general health and well-being.

Hormone imbalance is a complicated and varied disorder that can affect people at any point in their lives and for a variety of reasons. Understanding its causes, symptoms, and treatment options enables people to seek appropriate medical care, make informed lifestyle decisions, and strive for and maintain excellent hormonal health.

Common Hormone Imbalances: Thyroid Hormone Imbalance: Hypothyroidism (underactive thyroid) and hyperthyroidism (overactive thyroid) impact metabolism, energy levels, and weight.

- Sex Hormone Imbalance: Conditions such as polycystic ovarian syndrome (PCOS) in women and low testosterone in men can affect reproductive

systems, resulting in irregular menstrual cycles, infertility, and changes in sexual characteristics.
- Insulin Imbalance: Insulin resistance, which is commonly associated with obesity and sedentary lifestyles, hinders the body's capacity to regulate blood sugar levels, increasing the risk of type 2 diabetes and weight gain.
- Adrenal Hormone Imbalance: Disorders including Cushing's syndrome (high cortisol) and Addison's disease (low cortisol and aldosterone) have an impact on stress response, metabolism, and blood pressure management.

Hormone imbalance can cause a variety of symptoms, including: Symptoms may include weight gain, trouble reducing weight, fatigue, and low energy.
- Mood swings, anxiety, and despair
Symptoms may include irregular menstrual periods, infertility, changes in libido, and sexual function.
- Hair loss or rapid hair growth

- Sleep disorders.
- Digestive problems and appetite changes

Causes of Hormonal Imbalance
Hormone imbalance can result from a number of circumstances, including:

1. Dietary factors:
- Nutrient Deficiencies: A lack of key nutrients such as vitamins (e.g., vitamin D, vitamin B12) and minerals (e.g., zinc, magnesium) can impair hormone production and function.
- High Sugar and Processed Foods: A diet high in refined sugars and processed foods can cause insulin resistance and dysregulation of insulin and other metabolism-related hormones.

2. Lifestyle Choices:
- Lack of Physical Activity: A sedentary lifestyle and insufficient exercise might reduce insulin sensitivity, resulting in insulin resistance and hormonal imbalance.
- Sleep Deprivation: Inadequate

sleep or interrupted sleep patterns can interfere with hormone production, particularly growth hormone and cortisol, which alter metabolism, hunger, and stress responses.

3. Environmental Factors:

- Endocrine Disrupting Chemicals (EDCs): Exposure to chemicals from pesticides, plastics (e.g., BPA), household cleansers, and personal care products can disrupt hormone production and signaling. These substances can imitate hormones (estrogens), inhibit hormone receptors, or disrupt hormone metabolism.

- Heavy Metals: Exposure to heavy metals, including lead, mercury, and cadmium can impair hormone production and function.

4. Medical conditions and treatments:

- Chronic Illnesses: Chronic stress, autoimmune diseases, and inflammatory disorders may affect hormone balance.

- Medical Treatments: Radiation therapy, chemotherapy, and some drugs (such as corticosteroids and hormone therapies) can disrupt hormone production and regulation.

5. Psychological Factors:

- Chronic Stress: High cortisol levels can disturb hormones affecting metabolism, immunological function, and reproductive health.

- Mental Health Disorders: Depression and anxiety can disrupt hormone homeostasis by acting on the hypothalamic-pituitary-adrenal (HPA) axis and neurotransmitter systems.

6. Age-related Changes:

- During perimenopause and menopause, fluctuations in estrogen, progesterone, and other hormones can cause hormone imbalance symptoms such as hot flashes, mood swings, and weight gain.

- Andropause: In men, the age-related decline in testosterone levels (andropause) can cause weariness, decreased libido, and body composition changes.

7. Genetic Factors:

- Genetic predispositions can impact hormone production, receptor sensitivity, and metabolism, leading to hormonal imbalances such as insulin resistance, thyroid problems, and reproductive hormone abnormalities.

8. Pregnancy and Postpartum:
- Hormonal fluctuations during pregnancy and childbirth can cause illnesses such as gestational diabetes, postpartum depression, and thyroid function alterations.

9. Endocrine Gland Dysfunction:
- Disorders of hormone-producing glands such as the thyroid (hypothyroidism or hyperthyroidism) or the pancreas (diabetes mellitus).

Understanding the causes of hormonal imbalance highlights the complexity of hormonal regulation and the need to address lifestyle variables, environmental exposures, and medical illnesses that can affect hormone production and function. Managing hormone balance frequently necessitates a multifaceted approach that includes food, exercise, stress management, and medicinal interventions suited to specific requirements and circumstances.

Diagnosing and treating hormone imbalance often entails a medical history review, physical examination, and hormone level testing (blood or saliva).
- Treatment is based on the underlying cause and may involve lifestyle changes (diet, exercise, stress management), drugs (such as hormone replacement therapy or insulin sensitizers), and, in certain cases, surgical procedures (e.g., thyroidectomy).
- Acupuncture, herbal medicine, and nutritional supplementation are examples of integrative techniques that can help manage symptoms and promote hormonal balance.
Untreated hormone imbalances can cause chronic health issues like diabetes, cardiovascular disease, osteoporosis, and infertility.
- Hormonal variations can contribute to mood problems and

a lower quality of life, which may have an impact on psychological well-being. - Managing hormone balance is critical not just for symptom relief but also for overall health optimization and the prevention of long-term consequences.

Feeling weary and sleepy is a typical occurrence that can be caused by excessive physical activity, lack of sleep, improper eating habits, or a side effect of some medications. Although the majority of these factors may be managed and avoided, fatigue in the weeks preceding PMS and during your period may be caused by an underlying health problem.

Many women suffer from menorrhagia, sometimes known as heavy periods. Approximately one in every three women will seek therapy for the condition.

If excessive bleeding interferes with your daily life, don't ignore it; your body may be signaling you something is gravely wrong.

Extreme tiredness may be an underlying medical condition. Heavy monthly bleeding frequently causes women to feel weary, sometimes known as period fatigue. This is normal because estrogen levels drop around this time in your menstrual cycle. Your energy levels should return to normal after a few days, as your hormone levels begin to rise again. However, for other women, period fatigue and mood fluctuations might linger longer and be more severe. Some women may experience pre-menstrual symptoms, including feeling completely sluggish and unable to carry out basic activities, indicating a more serious condition.

This should be addressed because there could be a medical reason or underlying gynecological issues causing your low energy levels and lethargy during your period. You may be naturally weary during your periods or have anemia or an underactive thyroid. The main thing to remember is that you should never disregard severe menstrual   fatigue.

Premenstrual syndrome (PMS)
Before their menstruation, a few women will experience a series of symptoms in a regular order. Premenstrual syndrome refers to severe physical and emotional health changes that occur prior to the start of your period and last for a few days afterward. While some PMS symptoms are comparable to those felt after a period, their severity considerably disrupts daily life and causes physical and mental distress.

Period weariness is a symptom of premenstrual syndrome. Some people experience PMS symptoms before and during their period. These symptoms are caused by hormonal changes that occur around the time of menstruation.
More than 90% of people who get their periods report having PMS symptoms. Period fatigue

may be accompanied by the following PMS symptoms: Headache sleep issues, appetite changes, irritability, anxiety, depression, mood swings, crying bouts, period pain, and bloating.

Although the exact origin of premenstrual syndrome is unknown, research suggests that hormone changes, pre-existing mental health difficulties, and specific lifestyle circumstances are all important factors. Premenstrual dysphoric disorder refers to severe forms of premenstrual syndrome that require additional medical attention.

Some people experience a lack of energy or increased weariness just before or during their period. They may refer to these bouts as "period fatigue."

Causes

Although the exact origin of PMS is still debated, doctors believe it is caused by hormonal changes. The female ovaries generate the hormones estrogen and progesterone.

Estrogen production rises throughout the first half of the menstrual cycle and falls in the second half. Serotonin levels often decrease as estrogen levels fall. Low amounts of this neurotransmitter might cause depression and fatigue. Other probable reasons for period fatigue are:

Low iron: Heavy bleeding during menstruation might cause iron deficiency anemia. Without enough iron, the body cannot produce hemoglobin, which red blood cells require to deliver oxygen to the body's cells. Symptoms may include weakness and weariness. Food cravings: At times, a person may feel food cravings. Eating too much food may cause a spike and a subsequent drop in blood glucose levels. This dip may leave a person feeling lethargic and exhausted. Disrupted sleep: Period discomfort and mood changes might make it difficult to get asleep or stay asleep all night. The person may then feel sleepy and fatigued the next day.

Treatment

The following are some potential therapy options for period fatigue:

• nonsteroidal anti-inflammatory medications.

Nonsteroidal anti-inflammatory medicines (NSAIDs), such as ibuprofen, can help reduce pain and inflammation. If cramps are keeping a person awake, using an NSAID before bedtime may help them sleep more soundly. As a result, individuals may experience less fatigue the next day.

• Birth control pills. A doctor may prescribe birth control medications to help control hormone levels. They may prescribe taking the pills consecutively and skipping the placebo tablets or the pill-free week. This could help reduce hormonal changes, decreasing PMS symptoms.

• Supplements

The American College of Obstetricians and Gynecologists recommends taking 1,200 mg of calcium each day to help minimize physical and mental PMS symptoms.

Before starting any new supplement, a person should always consult with their doctor. Some supplements may interact with the person's existing drugs.

•   Antidepressants. In certain circumstances, doctors may prescribe antidepressants known as selective serotonin reuptake inhibitors (SSRIs) to treat both the mental and physical symptoms of PMS. Reducing these symptoms may make a person feel more rested and less exhausted, but a doctor should regularly supervise this treatment.
Examples of SSRIs are: Prozac (fluoxetine), Cipramil (citalopram), and Lustral (sertraline).

•   Home   Care
People can try the following measures at home to help decrease period fatigue:

- Adjusting the room temperature

A person's basal body temperature rises by roughly 0.5°C before their period, which can lead to poor or interrupted sleep. Lowering the room temperature somewhat may aid with comfort and sleep quality, resulting in less exhaustion the next day.

- Applying relaxing techniques. Some people may have difficulties falling asleep while on their period, which can contribute to increased weariness the following day.

- Sleeping difficulties can be caused by bodily aches and pains, as well as increased stress or anxiety. The following relaxation exercises can help relieve tension in the body and mind:

Practice mindfulness meditation and breathing exercises. Gentle exercise and massage. Taking a warm bath before bedtime.
Perform aerobic exercise.

A 2014 study looked at the

impact of aerobic exercise on 30 young women experiencing PMS symptoms. All subjects were given daily vitamin B6 and calcium tablets. Some also did aerobic activity three times each week for three months.

In comparison to the control group, people who exercised on a regular basis experienced much less period fatigue. Along with this came improvements in blood health, such as higher hemoglobin levels.
Trying alternative remedies. A 2014 meta-analysis found that acupuncture and several herbal therapies may help relieve PMS symptoms. According to the study, acupuncture and botanicals like ginkgo biloba reduced PMS symptoms by 50% or more compared to no treatment.

Chapter 3

Hormone levels fluctuate substantially with age and over time in both men and women, influencing numerous aspects of health and wellbeing. These alterations are impacted by puberty, reproductive cycles, age, and general physiological changes. Here's how hormone levels change throughout life for both genders:

In Women:

1. The puberty and reproductive years:
- Estrogen and Progesterone: During puberty, estrogen levels rise, causing the development of secondary sexual characteristics and the commencement of menstruation. Progesterone levels also rise, controlling the menstrual cycle and preparing the uterus for pregnancy.
- Menstrual Cycle: Estrogen and

progesterone levels change during the menstrual cycle, affecting mood, energy, and reproductive function.

2. Childbearing years:
- Pregnancy: Hormone levels, notably estrogen and progesterone, rise dramatically throughout pregnancy to aid fetal development and prepare the body for childbirth.
- Menopause Transition: Between the late 30s and early 50s, women go through perimenopause, which is characterized by a steady drop in estrogen and progesterone production, irregular monthly periods, and, eventually, menopause.

3. After menopause: - Estrogen Decline: Low estrogen levels can cause symptoms like hot flashes, vaginal dryness, and bone density abnormalities.
- Hormone Replacement Therapy (HRT): Some women may choose HRT to treat menopausal symptoms and lower their risk of osteoporosis and heart disease.

In   Men:

1. Puberty during the Adolescent Years:
- Testosterone: During puberty, testosterone levels rise, resulting in the development of male secondary sexual traits such as facial hair, a deeper voice, and muscle   gain.
- Sperm Production: Testosterone also influences sperm production and   reproductive   function.

2.   Adulthood: -   consistent Levels: Testosterone levels are normally   consistent   into adulthood,   supporting   libido, muscle mass, and bone density.
- Gradual Decline: Beginning around the age of 30, men's testosterone   production   may decrease by roughly 1% every year.

3.   Andropause   (male menopause):
- Symptoms: Some men may have symptoms related to low testosterone   levels,   including decreased   libido,   erectile dysfunction,   exhaustion,   and mood   changes.

- Health Risks: Low testosterone levels can raise the risk of osteoporosis, cardiovascular disease, and metabolic problems.

General Aging Effects:

Hormonal decline, especially growth hormone, affects metabolism, muscle mass, and overall vitality in both genders as they age.
- Hormone changes can lead to diminished energy, altered body composition (more body fat, less muscular mass), and lower bone density.

Age-related hormonal changes can increase the risk of chronic illnesses such as osteoporosis, cardiovascular disease, and metabolic syndrome.
- Maintaining a healthy lifestyle, which includes regular physical activity, balanced nutrition, and stress management, can help reduce the effects of age-related hormone changes.

Understanding these age-related hormone changes emphasizes the significance of regular health monitoring, lifestyle changes, and, when needed, medical interventions to maintain hormonal balance and overall well-being throughout life.

Tips for Postmenopausal Women
Nutrition After Menopause

The key to remaining youthful and energetic after menopause is proper nutrition and regular physical activity.
Your nutritional needs alter as you get older. Before menopause, you should consume approximately 1,000 mg of calcium every day. Following menopause, you should consume up to 1,200 mg of calcium each day.

Vitamin D has a crucial role in calcium absorption and bone growth. Vitamin D can significantly reduce the risk of spinal fractures. However, consuming too much calcium or vitamin D might result in kidney stones, constipation, or abdominal pain, particularly if you have renal problems.

The importance of exercising after menopause

Many women gain weight following menopause. This could be due to diminishing estrogen levels. Raising your level of activity will help you prevent gaining weight. Regular exercise benefits the heart and bones, aids in weight management, and can enhance your attitude. Women who are physically inactive are more likely to develop heart disease, obesity, high blood pressure, diabetes, and osteoporosis. Sedentary women may also experience persistent back pain, sleeplessness, poor circulation, weakened muscles, and depression.

Aerobic activities, including walking, jogging, swimming, biking, and dancing, can help prevent some of these issues. It also helps to boost HDL cholesterol levels, or "good" cholesterol. Weight-bearing exercises like walking and jogging, as well as modest weight training, can help improve bone mass. Moderate exercise helps postmenopausal women maintain bone mass in the spine and avoid fractures.

Exercise also improves mood. The brain produces hormones known as endorphins. The improved mood lasts several hours. It also aids the body in combating stress.

Always consult your healthcare provider before beginning an exercise regimen, especially if you have been inactive. Your healthcare practitioner can suggest the ideal exercise regimen for you.

Sex after menopause.

Some women lose interest in sex during or after menopause. Menopause symptoms, such as drier vaginal tissues and reduced estrogen levels, may contribute to a decline in sexual interest. Estrogen creams and tablets, however, can help restore genital suppleness and secretions. Personal lubricants may also make sex more enjoyable.

Women who experience erratic periods throughout perimenopause should continue to use some sort of birth control. Consult your healthcare practitioner about which type of birth control is best for you.

Maintaining health after menopause.

These suggestions will help you live a healthy life after menopause. For further information, please contact your healthcare provider.

• Before deciding on hormone replacement therapy, talk to your doctor about the risks and advantages.

• Do not smoke. Smoking is a significant risk factor for cardiovascular disease.

• Exercise regularly. Even modest activity, such as walking for half an hour three times each week, is good.

• Maintain a healthy weight by following a balanced, low-sugar diet.

• Manage high blood pressure with medication or lifestyle modifications. This will help lower your risk of heart disease.

• Reduce your stress levels with relaxation techniques or frequent exercise.

Hormone growth that affects your weight

Several hormones influence metabolism, hunger, fat storage, and energy expenditure, all of which contribute significantly to weight regulation. Understanding how these hormones work can reveal how they affect body weight:

1. Insulin: - The pancreas produces insulin, which controls blood sugar levels by enabling glucose uptake into cells for energy and storage.
- Effect on Weight: Insulin encourages fat storage, particularly when blood sugar levels are high. Insulin resistance

occurs when cells become less responsive to insulin, resulting in chronically increased insulin levels and weight accumulation, particularly around the abdomen.

2. Leptin: - Role: Fat cells create leptin, which signals the brain to reduce appetite and boost energy expenditure.
- Weight Impact: Leptin resistance, or the brain's inability to respond appropriately to leptin signals, can result in overeating and weight gain. Obese people frequently have high amounts of leptin but are less sensitive to its effects.

3. Ghrelin: - The stomach produces ghrelin, which stimulates appetite.
- Effect on Weight: Ghrelin levels rise before meals and fall after eating. Imbalances in ghrelin production or sensitivity can increase hunger and contribute to weight gain.

4. Cortisol: - The adrenal glands create cortisol in reaction to stress, which regulates metabolism, blood sugar levels,

and immunological responses.
- Effect on Weight: Chronic stress can cause high cortisol levels, which can increase hunger and encourage fat formation, particularly visceral fat around the abdomen.

5. Thyroid Hormones: - Thyroid hormones control metabolism and energy expenditure in the body.
- Effect on Weight: Hypothyroidism (low thyroid hormone levels) can cause slower metabolism and weight gain, whereas hyperthyroidism (excess thyroid hormone) can accelerate metabolism and cause weight loss.

6. Estrogen and progesterone (in women):
- Role: Estrogen and progesterone regulate reproductive activities as well as metabolism and fat distribution.
- Effect on Weight: Fluctuations in estrogen and progesterone levels during the menstrual cycle, pregnancy, and menopause might affect women's appetite, fat storage, and weight management.

7. Testosterone (for men):
- involvement: While testosterone is well known for its involvement in male sexual development and reproductive function, it also influences metabolism and muscle mass.
- Effect on Weight: Low testosterone levels in men can lead to decreased muscle mass, increased body fat, and possibly weight gain.

Understanding how these hormones interact and how they affect weight regulation can help people make informed decisions about lifestyle choices such as nutrition, exercise, stress management, and sleep, which will help them maintain healthy hormone levels and weight. When necessary, medical interventions can help balance these hormones and help you achieve and maintain your best health and well-being.

Balanced testosterone and estrogen levels for increased vitality

Achieving a healthy testosterone/estrogen ratio is critical for energy and overall health, especially as we age. In addition to their primary involvement in reproductive health, both hormones play important roles in a variety of physiological functions. Here's how balancing testosterone and estrogen can improve vitality:

Testosterone:

1. Men's Role: - Preventing Estrogen Dominance: As men age, testosterone levels may decrease while estrogen levels remain stable or rise due to testosterone conversion to estrogen in adipose tissue. This imbalance, known as estrogen dominance, can cause symptoms such as weight gain (especially in the abdomen), exhaustion, and a decrease in libido. - Increasing Testosterone Production: Lifestyle factors such as regular exercise, proper sleep, and a well-balanced diet rich in nutrients like zinc and vitamin D can help boost testosterone production.

- Medical Intervention: In some circumstances, testosterone replacement therapy (TRT) may be prescribed under medical supervision to restore testosterone levels and boost vitality.
- Muscle Mass and Strength: Testosterone promotes muscle growth and maintenance, which improves physical strength and vitality.
- Bone Density: It promotes bone health and density while lowering the risk of osteoporosis.
- Libido and Sexual Function: Testosterone is essential for sexual desire (libido), erectile function, and general sexual health.
- Mood and Energy: It can improve your mood, energy level, and general sense of well-being.

2. Women's Role: - Maintaining Hormonal Balance: During perimenopause and menopause,

estrogen and testosterone levels fall. Balancing these hormones with hormone replacement therapy (HRT) or natural methods can help control symptoms and promote vitality.
- Lifestyle Factors: Regular exercise, stress management, and a nutritious diet can help to balance hormones and improve overall vitality.
- Consultation with a healthcare professional: Women who are experiencing symptoms of hormone imbalance should speak with a healthcare professional about treatment choices and monitoring.
- Energy and vigor: Testosterone helps women maintain their energy and vigor.
- Bone Health: It supports bone density and lowers the risk of osteoporosis.
- Libido: Testosterone is responsible for sexual desire and arousal in women.

Estrogen:

1. The Role of Women:
- Bone Health: Estrogen helps preserve bone density and lowers

the risk of osteoporosis.
- Cardiovascular Health: It promotes healthy cholesterol levels and improves cardiovascular function.
- Brain Function: Estrogen influences cognitive function, memory, and mood control.
- Skin Health: It improves skin elasticity and moisture retention.

Lifestyle strategies for hormone balance:

- Regular Exercise: Aerobic and resistance activities can help boost testosterone production and balance hormone levels.
- Healthy Diet: Eating a well-balanced diet rich in nutrients such as lean proteins, healthy fats, fruits, and vegetables promotes overall hormonal health.
- Stress Management: Chronic stress can disrupt hormone balance. Mindfulness, yoga, and relaxation exercises are all effective stress-management techniques.
- Adequate Sleep: Proper sleep is necessary for hormone

production and overall health.

Understanding the roles of testosterone and estrogen, as well as implementing lifestyle choices to support hormonal balance, can help people maintain physical and mental well-being and enjoy a greater quality of life as they age

Chapter 4

Roles of hormone in the reproductive health of women

Hormones are important in women's reproductive health because they regulate menstrual cycles, promote fertility, and facilitate conception. These hormones are produced by many glands and tissues throughout the body, and their coordinated action ensures that the female reproductive system functions properly. Here are the main hormones involved, as well as their functions:

Estrogen:

Menstrual Cycle Regulation:
- During the first part of the menstrual cycle, the ovaries (especially the follicles therein) generate estrogen, which stimulates the growth and development of the uterine lining (endometrium).
- It increases endometrial cell proliferation in preparation for embryo implantation.

Secondary sex characteristics:
- Estrogen is responsible for the development of secondary sexual traits during puberty, including breast development, hip widening, and pubic and axillary hair growth.

Regulation of gonadotropins:
- Estrogen inhibits the release of gonadotropins (FSH and LH) from the pituitary gland. This helps to control the timing of ovulation and the menstrual cycle.

Progesterone:

The menstrual cycle is regulated:
-    Progesterone, which is

predominantly produced by the corpus luteum (a structure created from the ovarian follicle after ovulation) and then by the placenta during pregnancy, is essential for regulating the menstrual cycle.
- It prepares the endometrium for the implantation of a fertilized egg and helps to maintain the uterine lining throughout early pregnancy.

Pregnancy Support:
- During pregnancy, progesterone helps to regulate the uterine environment, limiting contractions that could result in preterm labor.
- It also promotes fetal growth and development while preparing the breasts for milk production.

Follicle stimulating hormone (FSH) and luteinizing hormone (LH):

Ovulation Induction:
- The pituitary gland releases FSH and LH in response to hypothalamic signals. FSH promotes the growth and maturity of ovarian follicles,

which contain developing eggs.
- LH causes ovulation, or the release of a mature egg from the ovarian follicles. This often occurs in the middle of the menstrual cycle.

Human Chorionic Gonadotropin (HCG):

Pregnancy detection:
- The placenta produces HCG immediately after the embryo has been implanted in the uterine lining.
- It helps to preserve the corpus luteum, which produces progesterone throughout the early stages of pregnancy.
- HCG is a hormone found in pregnancy tests that acts as an indicator of pregnancy.

Prolactin:

Role in Breastfeeding
- The pituitary gland produces prolactin, which increases milk production (lactation) in the mammary glands of the breasts.
- It works with oxytocin to promote milk ejection (letdown)

during   nursing.

Oxytocin:

Labor and Milk Ejection:
- The pituitary gland also produces oxytocin, which plays an important role in uterine contractions during labor and delivery.
- It also accelerates the milk ejection reflex (letdown) during breastfeeding, which promotes baby nutrition.

Thyroid Hormones (T3, T4):

Fertility Regulation:
- Thyroid hormones affect reproductive health by regulating menstrual cycle regularity and ovarian function.
- Abnormal thyroid hormone levels (hypothyroidism or hyperthyroidism) might affect fertility and pregnancy outcomes.

Role in Menopause:

Transition and Symptoms:
- During menopause, estrogen and progesterone levels drop, resulting in the cessation of

monthly periods and symptoms like hot flashes, vaginal dryness, and mood swings.
- Hormone replacement therapy (HRT) can help relieve menopausal symptoms while also lowering the long-term risks of osteoporosis and cardiovascular disease.

In summary, hormones have complex and important functions in women's reproductive health, regulating menstrual cycles, promoting fertility, aiding pregnancy, and altering secondary sexual traits. Understanding these hormone actions is critical for controlling reproductive health throughout life and resolving any hormone-related disorders that may occur.

Women's hormonal issues during childbirth
A healthy pregnancy requires a proper hormonal balance. Hormones serve as the body's chemical messengers, transmitting information and feeding back responses between tissues and organs. Hormones

circulate throughout the body, typically via the blood, and bind to proteins on cells known as receptors, much like a key fits a lock or a hand fits a glove. In reaction, the target tissue or organ operates in such a way that the pregnancy is sustained. Initially, the ovaries, and subsequently the placenta, are the primary makers of pregnancy-related hormones that are required to create and sustain the proper conditions for a healthy pregnancy.

The initial stages of pregnancy Following fertilization, a new embryo must announce its presence to the mother, allowing her body to detect the onset of pregnancy. When an egg is fertilized, it travels through the female reproductive canal before implanting into the womb roughly 9 days later, releasing a hormone known as human chorionic gonadotrophin. This hormone enters the maternal bloodstream, allowing the mother to detect the embryo and begin to prepare her body for pregnancy. Throughout pregnancy, this hormone is produced at enormous levels.

Human chorionic gonadotrophin can be detected in urine as early as 7-9 days after fertilization and is utilized in the majority of over-the-counter pregnancy tests. It is partly responsible for the frequent urination that many pregnant women suffer during the first trimester. This is because increased levels of human chorionic gonadotropin encourage more blood to flow to the pelvic area and kidneys, allowing the kidneys to remove waste more quickly than before pregnancy. Human chorionic gonadotrophin travels through the mother's bloodstream to the ovaries, where it regulates the levels of the pro-pregnancy hormones estrogen and progesterone.

The role of progesterone and estrogen in pregnancy

High levels of progesterone are necessary during pregnancy, with levels gradually increasing until the baby's delivery. During the first few weeks of pregnancy, progesterone produced by the corpus luteum (a transient endocrine gland in the ovaries) is adequate to maintain pregnancy. At this early stage, progesterone has many diverse activities that are critical to the establishment of pregnancy, including:

• Increasing blood supply to the womb by encouraging the expansion of existing blood vessels.

• stimulating glands in the womb lining (the endometrium) to create nourishment for the developing embryo.

• stimulating endometrial growth and thickening, resulting in the decidua (a distinct organ that enables placental attachment) and embryo implantation.

• Contributing to the development of the placenta. As the placenta matures and develops, it gains the ability to create hormones. The cells that make up the placenta, known as trophoblasts, can convert cholesterol from the mother's bloodstream into progesterone. Between weeks 6 and 9 of pregnancy, the placenta replaces the ovaries as the primary generator of progesterone. Progesterone serves a variety of tasks during mid- to late pregnancy, including:

• It is critical for proper fetal development.

• Preventing the womb muscles from contracting until labor begins.

• Avoid lactation (breastfeeding) until after pregnancy.

• Strengthening the pelvic wall muscles to prepare for labor. Although progesterone is the dominant hormone during pregnancy, estrogen is also quite significant. Many of progesterone's actions rely on estrogen, and estrogen actually stimulates progesterone production from the placenta. Initially, the corpus luteum of the ovaries produces and releases estrogen. As the pregnancy progresses, the foetal adrenal glands create androgens, which are subsequently transported to the placenta and transformed into the hormone oestriol (an estrogen commonly used to assess foetal health throughout pregnancy) and other oestrogens. Oestriol levels rise continuously until birth and have numerous impacts, including:

• Managing, regulating, and increasing the production of other pregnancy hormones.

• Ensures proper development of several fetal organs, including the lungs, liver, and kidneys.

• stimulating placental growth and function.

• Promoting maternal breast tissue growth (in conjunction with progesterone) and preparing the mother for nursing.

Other hormones generated by the placenta

The placenta also generates

additional hormones, such as human placental lactogen and corticotropin-releasing hormone. Human placental lactogen's function is not fully understood, although it is assumed to encourage mammary gland growth in preparation for breastfeeding. It is also thought to help control the mother's metabolism by boosting the amount of nutrients in her blood that the fetus can use. Corticotropin-releasing hormone is hypothesized to control the length of pregnancy and fetal development. For example, when pregnant women are stressed, especially in the first trimester, the placenta produces more corticotrophin-releasing hormones. There is a valid reason for this. Corticotropin-releasing hormone suppresses the mother's immune system in the early stages of pregnancy, preventing it from attacking the baby. Later in pregnancy, it enhances blood flow between the placenta and the fetus. Corticotrophin-releasing hormone levels peak in the latter weeks of pregnancy, coinciding with a significant increase in cortisol levels. The increase in corticotropin-releasing hormone and cortisol may help the fetal organs mature right before labor begins, influencing the date of birth via a 'late-term cortisol surge'. This prenatal cortisol increase has also been linked to more attentive maternal behavior in both animals and women. It is supposed to be an adaptive response that causes a greater love for their infant's bodily odors, hence enhancing the mother-baby bond.

Pregnancy hormones can cause side effects.

High levels of progesterone and estrogen are essential for a healthy pregnancy, but they are frequently the source of certain common unpleasant side effects in the mother, particularly since they act on the brain. Until the mother's body adjusts to the greater amounts of these hormones, mood swings are typical. The majority of women will suffer morning sickness, which is characterized by nausea at any time of day and can progress to vomiting. The specific origin of morning sickness is unknown; however, it is most likely caused by a sudden surge in estrogen, progesterone, and human chorionic gonadotropin, or a drop in thyroid stimulating hormone (which is structurally identical to human chorionic gonadotrophin). However, it is most likely caused by a combination of these hormonal changes. Morning sickness typically begins about weeks 5–6 of pregnancy and normally diminishes by weeks 12–16, though some women experience it throughout pregnancy and/or have more severe forms of morning sickness.

During the first trimester, many women have pelvic and lower back pain and discomfort. This is primarily due to the hormone relaxin. Relaxin is detected between weeks 7 and 10, and it is generated throughout pregnancy. This hormone relaxes the mother's muscles, joints, and ligaments to allow room for the growing baby. Relaxin's actions are largely focused in the pelvic region, therefore, softening the pelvic joints can often cause pain in that location. Softer pelvic joints can also reduce stability, and some women may find it difficult to balance.

Although difficult and annoying at times, all of these side effects often diminish or disappear by the end of the first trimester.

Hormones During Labor The specific events that preceded the onset of labor are still unknown. Before the baby can be born, two things must happen: the muscles in the womb and abdominal wall must contract, and the cervix must soften or ripen, allowing the baby to pass from the womb to the outside world.

The hormone oxytocin has an important function in labor. Oxytocin, also known as the 'love hormone', is linked to feelings of connection and motherhood. This is also true for prolactin, another hormone that is released during delivery. If labor needs to be induced (started artificially), oxytocin or a synthetic oxytocin counterpart is frequently used to 'kick-start' the process. When labor begins, oxytocin levels rise, forcing the womb and abdominal muscles to contract on a regular basis.

The cervix must dilate (open) to approximately 10 cm for the baby to pass through. Oxytocin, coupled with other hormones, causes the cervix to soften, resulting in sequential dilation during labor. Oxytocin, together with high levels of estrogen, stimulates the release of a group of hormones known as prostaglandins, which may contribute to cervix softening. During labor, relaxation levels rise dramatically. This promotes the lengthening and softening of the cervix, as well as the softening and expansion of the mother's lower pelvic region, thereby facilitating the baby's delivery.

As the intensity of labor contractions increases, natural

pain relieving chemicals are released. Beta-endorphins, like morphine, work on the same receptors in the brain. In addition to pain relief, they can make the mother feel elated and happy. As birth approaches, the mother's body produces high amounts of adrenaline and noradrenaline, also known as 'fight or flight' hormones. A quick burst of these hormones soon before birth allows the woman to feel energized and have several very intense contractions, which aid in the delivery of the baby.

Hormones following labor
When the baby is born, oxytocin continues to compress the womb to limit blood flow and lessen the risk of hemorrhage, as well as to aid in the detachment of the placenta (which is delivered shortly thereafter). Oxytocin and prolactin levels in the blood are extremely high, promoting maternal-fetal attachment. Skin-to-skin and eye contact between mother and infant enhance the release of oxytocin and prolactin, which further promotes bonding. Many moms report feeling

euphoric immediately after labor due to the effects of oxytocin, prolactin, and beta-endorphins.

Women can breastfeed approximately four months into their pregnancy, but high levels of progesterone and estrogen hinder milk production. After the placenta is delivered at birth, the mother's blood levels of progesterone and estrogen fall, allowing her to make the first meal of colostrum, a high-density milk with more protein, minerals, and fat-soluble vitamins (A and K) than mature milk, which is produced later. When a baby suckles, the pituitary gland releases oxytocin and prolactin, which travel through the mother's blood to the breast. Prolactin boosts milk production, while oxytocin stimulates milk delivery to the nipple. These hormones not only promote bonding but also help with milk release and production. Mature milk, which nourishes the baby and encourages sleep, begins to be produced around four days after birth.

Effects of hormonal imbalances on female health. Hormone imbalance in women can have a substantial impact on many facets of health, including physical, emotional, and reproductive health. The effects vary according to which hormones are unbalanced and how severe the imbalance is. Here are some common effects of hormonal imbalances on female health:

1. Menstrual irregularities:
- Hormone imbalances, especially those involving estrogen and progesterone, can cause irregular menstrual cycles, such as skipped periods, prolonged bleeding, or heavy periods.
- Polycystic ovarian syndrome (PCOS), characterized by high testosterone levels and insulin resistance, can impair ovulation and monthly regularity.

2. Fertility Issues:
- Hormonal disruptions can reduce fertility by influencing ovulation, egg quality, and the

uterine environment required for implantation.
- Infertility can be caused by luteal phase defects (inadequate progesterone production), thyroid abnormalities, and high prolactin levels (hyperprolactinemia).

3. Menopause Symptoms:
- Lower levels of estrogen and progesterone during perimenopause and menopause can cause symptoms like hot flashes, nocturnal sweats, mood swings, vaginal dryness, and decreased libido.
- Hormone replacement therapy (HRT) may be used to treat these symptoms and lower the long-term health concerns associated with hormonal decline.

4. Bone Health:
- Estrogen helps to maintain bone density and strength. A decrease in estrogen levels, such as during menopause, raises the risk of osteoporosis and fracture.
- Hormonal abnormalities that interfere with calcium metabolism or vitamin D absorption can have an influence on bone health.

5. Metabolic and Weight Issues:
- Insulin resistance, which is frequently associated with disorders such as PCOS, can cause weight gain, particularly in the abdomen, and increase the risk of type 2 diabetes.
- Thyroid hormone imbalances (hypothyroidism or hyperthyroidism) can disrupt metabolism, causing weight fluctuations, lethargy, and other symptoms.

6. Mood and mental health:
- Hormonal variations, such as those associated with the menstrual cycle or perimenopause, can have an impact on mood swings, irritability, anxiety, and sadness.
- Estrogen is thought to have neuroprotective properties, and its loss during menopause may lead to cognitive abnormalities and mood swings.

7. Skin and hair changes:
- Hormonal imbalances can have an impact on skin health, causing acne, dryness, and excessive oil production.

- Androgen level changes, such as increased testosterone, can lead to hirsutism (excess face and body hair) or hair loss (androgenetic alopecia).

8. Cardiovascular Health:
- Estrogen promotes healthy cholesterol levels and improves cardiovascular function. Following menopause, decreased estrogen levels may raise the risk of heart disease and stroke.

9. Breast Health:
- Hormonal imbalances, particularly high estrogen levels in comparison to progesterone, may raise the risk of breast cancer.
- Hormonal shifts during the menstrual cycle might also influence breast discomfort and sensitivity.

Managing Hormonal Imbalance
Managing hormone imbalance necessitates a multifaceted strategy that tackles the underlying causes, symptoms, and general health of the

individual. Many tactics and factors for properly managing hormone imbalance are listed below:

1. Medical Examination and Diagnosis:
- Consultation with a Healthcare Provider: Seek advice from a hormone expert, such as a primary care physician, endocrinologist, or gynecologist.
- Hormone Testing: Test your hormone levels using blood tests, saliva tests, or other diagnostic instruments to find any imbalances.

2. Lifestyle modifications:
- Healthy Diet: Eat a well-balanced diet rich in whole foods, including fruits and vegetables, lean proteins, healthy fats, and complex carbohydrates. Avoid too much sugar, refined carbs, and processed foods.
- Regular Physical Activity: Exercise regularly, such as aerobics and strength training, to promote metabolism, hormone production, and overall health.
- Stress Management: To reduce

cortisol levels and promote hormone balance, try stress-reduction practices like mindfulness meditation, deep breathing exercises, yoga, or spending time in nature.
- Adequate Sleep: Aim for 7-9 hours of sleep per night to support hormone control, cellular repair, and overall wellness.

3. Nutritional Support:
- Consider taking supplements that help with hormone balance, such as vitamin D, magnesium, omega-3 fatty acids, and adaptogenic herbs like ashwagandha or rhodiola. However, before starting any supplements, contact a healthcare provider.
- Limit Alcohol and Caffeine: Avoid consuming alcohol and caffeine, which can disrupt hormone levels and have a bad impact on sleep and stress.

4. Hormone Replacement Therapy:
- For menopause, hormone

replacement therapy (HRT) may be administered to address menopausal symptoms such as hot flashes, night sweats, vaginal dryness, and mood swings. It usually contains estrogen, with or without progesterone.
- For Other Conditions: In cases of severe hormonal shortage or imbalance (e.g., hypothyroidism, adrenal insufficiency), hormone replacement therapy under medical supervision may be required.

5. Medication and treatments:
- Specific Conditions: Depending on the underlying cause of hormone imbalance (e.g., thyroid problems, PCOS), drugs such as thyroid hormone replacement, insulin sensitizers (for insulin resistance), or oral contraceptives (for hormonal management) may be recommended.
- Bioidentical Hormones: Some people choose bioidentical hormone therapy, which uses hormones that are chemically identical to those produced naturally in the body. This technique should be explored

with a healthcare professional.

6. Behavioral and Psychological Support:
- Counseling or Therapy: If hormone imbalance is harming your mental health or relationships, you should seek counseling or therapy to address emotional well-being, stress management, and coping skills.
- Support Groups: Joining support groups or online forums can provide emotional support as well as practical advice from people who are dealing with similar hormone-related issues.

7. Regular Monitoring and Adjustments:
- Follow-up consultations: Schedule regular follow-up consultations with your doctor to monitor hormone levels, review therapy efficacy, and make any required changes to your management plan.
- Self-awareness: Monitor changes in symptoms, mood, energy levels, and overall well-being. Keeping a journal can help you recognize patterns,

triggers, and areas for progress.

8. Education Resources:
- Stay Informed: Learn about hormone health, including their roles, typical imbalances, and treatment choices. Medical practitioners, trustworthy websites, and health groups are all reliable sources.

9. Holistic approaches:
- Complementary Therapies: Look into alternative treatments, including acupuncture, chiropractic care, herbal medicine, and homeopathy. These can help with hormone balance and overall wellness, but their effectiveness varies, so talk with a healthcare expert.

Understanding the effects of hormone imbalance on female health emphasizes the importance of taking preventive measures and seeking medical help if you have symptoms or concerns about hormonal swings. Early intervention and individualized treatment strategies can help reduce the consequences of hormone imbalance while also improving general health and quality of life. Managing hormone imbalance necessitates an individualized approach based on individual needs, health history, and hormone levels. Collaboration with healthcare experts, sticking to treatment programs, and making proactive lifestyle changes are essential for establishing hormone balance and improving overall health and quality of life.

Chapter 5

Hormone balance diet

A hormone-balancing diet focuses on consuming nutrient-dense foods that support hormone production, regulation, and overall health. Here are some key principles and food recommendations for a hormone-balancing diet:

1. **Balance Macronutrients:**

• **Proteins**: Lean Protein is essential for hormone synthesis and tissue repair. Such as:

- Chicken Breast: A lean source of protein that provides amino acids necessary for hormone production and tissue repair.
- Turkey: Another lean protein option that supports muscle health and overall metabolism.
- Legumes: Beans, lentils, and chickpeas are plant-based sources of protein, fiber, and minerals like zinc and iron, important for hormone balance.
• **Healthy Fats:** Opt for sources of healthy fats:
- Avocado: Rich in monounsaturated fats and potassium, which support cardiovascular health and hormone production.
- Nuts and Seeds: Almonds, walnuts, chia seeds, flaxseeds, and hemp seeds provide omega-3 fatty acids and zinc, essential for hormone synthesis and anti-inflammatory effects.
- Olive Oil: Contains monounsaturated fats and antioxidants, beneficial for heart health and reducing inflammation.
- Fatty Fish: Salmon, mackerel, trout, and sardines are rich in omega-3 fatty acids, which

support brain health, reduce inflammation, and promote hormone balance.

• **Complex Carbohydrates:** Choose whole grains (e.g., quinoa, brown rice, oats), fruits, and vegetables. These provide fiber and essential nutrients without causing rapid blood sugar spikes.

- Quinoa: A complete protein source rich in fiber, B vitamins, and minerals such as magnesium and zinc, which support energy production and hormone balance.

- Brown Rice: Provides complex carbohydrates for sustained energy and B vitamins essential for hormone metabolism.

- Oats: High in soluble fiber and beta-glucan, which promote digestive health and help regulate blood sugar levels.

2. **Include Phytonutrients and Antioxidants:**

• **Colorful Vegetables:** Consume a variety of colorful vegetables such as leafy greens, bell peppers, broccoli, carrots, and tomatoes. These are rich in antioxidants and phytonutrients that support overall health and hormone balance.

- Leafy Greens: Spinach, kale, Swiss chard, and collard greens are rich in vitamins (such as A, C, K) and minerals (like magnesium and calcium) that support overall health and hormone balance.

-       Cruciferous Vegetables: Broccoli, cauliflower, Brussels sprouts, and cabbage contain compounds like indole-3-carbinol and sulforaphane that help metabolize and balance estrogen levels.

- Bell Peppers: High in vitamin C and antioxidants, which support immune function and reduce oxidative stress.

-       Berries: Blueberries, strawberries, raspberries, and other berries are packed with antioxidants that help combat oxidative stress and inflammation.

3. **Supportive Herbs and Spices:**

- Turmeric: Contains curcumin, which has anti-inflammatory properties and may help balance hormones.

- Cinnamon: Helps regulate blood sugar levels, which is

important for insulin sensitivity and hormone balance.
- Ginger: Supports digestion and has anti-inflammatory effects.
4. **Fruits:**
- Citrus Fruits: Oranges, grapefruits, lemons, and limes are high in vitamin C, which supports immune function and collagen production.
- Bananas: Rich in potassium and B vitamins, which support nervous system function and energy metabolism.
5. **Probiotic-Rich Foods:**
- Yogurt: Contains probiotics that support gut health and digestion, which is essential for hormone metabolism and overall health.
- Kefir: A fermented dairy product rich in probiotics and calcium, which supports bone health and gut microbiota balance.
6. **Foods Rich in Specific Nutrients:**
- Zinc: Found in seafood, poultry, beans, nuts, and seeds. Zinc is crucial for the production of several hormones, including insulin and thyroid hormones.

- Magnesium: Found in spinach, almonds, avocado, and legumes. Magnesium supports hormone regulation and helps manage stress.
- Vitamin D: Found in fatty fish (e.g., salmon, mackerel), egg yolks, and fortified foods. Adequate vitamin D levels are important for hormonal balance.

7. **Others:**
- Green Tea: Contains catechins, antioxidants that support metabolism and may help reduce inflammation and promote weight loss.
- Dark Chocolate: Provides flavonoids and antioxidants that support heart health and may improve mood and hormone balance in moderation.

Explanation of Benefits:
- Omega-3 Fatty Acids: Found in fatty fish, nuts, and seeds, omega-3s reduce inflammation, support brain health, and may help regulate hormones like insulin and leptin.
- Fiber: Found in fruits, vegetables, and whole grains, fiber promotes digestive health, helps regulate blood sugar levels, and supports weight

management, all of which contribute to hormone balance.

- Antioxidants: Found in colorful fruits and vegetables, antioxidants protect cells from oxidative stress, reduce inflammation, and support overall health, including hormone balance.

- Vitamins and Minerals: Essential for hormone synthesis and metabolism, vitamins (such as B vitamins, vitamin D, and vitamin C) and minerals (such as zinc, magnesium, and selenium) play critical roles in supporting hormone production, energy metabolism, and overall well-being.

8. **Hydration:**

- Drink plenty of water throughout the day to support overall health and hormone balance. Herbal teas can also be a good option.

9. **Meal Timing and Portion Control:**

- Regular Meals: Aim for balanced meals throughout the day to maintain stable blood sugar levels and support hormone regulation.

- Portion Control: Avoid overeating and practice mindful eating to support digestion and metabolic health.

Sample Hormone-Balancing Meal Plan:

- Breakfast: Overnight oats with chia seeds, berries, and a sprinkle of nuts; or a spinach and mushroom omelet with whole grain toast.
- Lunch: Grilled chicken salad with mixed greens, avocado, tomatoes, and olive oil dressing; or quinoa with roasted vegetables and a side of grilled fish.
- Snack: Greek yogurt with a handful of almonds and a drizzle of honey; or carrot sticks with hummus.
- Dinner: Baked salmon with quinoa and steamed broccoli; or stir-fried tofu with vegetables in a ginger-turmeric sauce.

Important Considerations:

- Individual Needs: The ideal diet for hormone balance may vary depending on individual health conditions, hormonal imbalances, and dietary preferences. Consult with a healthcare provider or registered dietitian for personalized recommendations.

- Consistency: Adopting a hormone-balancing diet is most effective when combined with regular physical activity, stress management techniques, and adequate sleep.

By focusing on nutrient-dense foods, supporting hormone production and regulation, and avoiding or limiting foods that disrupt hormonal balance, individuals can support overall health and well-being through diet.

Incorporating these hormone-balancing foods into a well-rounded diet can support hormone production, metabolism, and overall health. It's important to maintain a balanced approach to nutrition, personalized to individual needs and health goals, while consulting with a healthcare provider or registered dietitian for personalized advice.

Foods to avoid

Maintaining hormone balance involves not only consuming beneficial foods but also avoiding or minimizing certain foods that can disrupt hormone production, regulation, and overall health. Here's an explanation of foods to avoid for hormone balance:

1. **Refined Carbohydrates and Sugars:**
- White Bread and Pasta: These are high in refined carbohydrates that can cause rapid spikes in blood sugar levels, leading to insulin resistance over time. Insulin resistance disrupts hormone balance, particularly insulin and leptin, which regulate metabolism and appetite.
- Sugary Foods and Beverages: Candies, pastries, sugary drinks, and desserts contribute to inflammation, weight gain, and insulin spikes, negatively impacting hormone levels.

2. **Trans Fats and Unhealthy Fats:**
- Hydrogenated Oils: Found in processed foods, margarine, and baked goods, trans fats increase inflammation and interfere with hormone synthesis and function.
- Processed Meats: Hot dogs, sausages, and bacon often contain unhealthy fats and

additives that can disrupt hormone balance and increase inflammation.

3. **Excessive Caffeine and Alcohol:**

- Caffeine: While moderate coffee consumption may have health benefits, excessive caffeine intake can disrupt cortisol levels and affect sleep patterns, leading to adrenal fatigue and hormonal imbalances.

- Alcohol: Excessive alcohol consumption can impair liver function, which is crucial for hormone metabolism and detoxification. It can also disrupt estrogen and testosterone balance.

4. **Soy Products (in some cases):**

- Processed Soy Products: Some soy products, especially highly processed ones like soy protein isolate or soybean oil, contain phytoestrogens (plant-based compounds with estrogen-like effects) that can interfere with natural hormone production and balance in some individuals.

5. **Dairy Products (in some cases):**

- Conventional Dairy: Some dairy products may contain hormones and antibiotics that can disrupt endocrine function in sensitive individuals. Additionally, lactose intolerance or sensitivity to dairy proteins can cause inflammation and digestive issues that may indirectly impact hormone balance.

6. **Artificial Sweeteners and Additives:**

- Aspartame, Sucralose, Saccharin: Found in diet sodas, sugar-free products, and some packaged foods, artificial sweeteners can disrupt gut microbiota and metabolism, potentially affecting hormone balance.

- Food Additives: Preservatives, colorings, and flavor enhancers in processed foods can contain chemicals that disrupt hormone signaling and metabolism.

7. **High Mercury Fish:**

- Large Predatory Fish: Swordfish, shark, king mackerel, and tilefish may contain high levels of mercury, which can interfere with hormone production and neurological function if consumed in excess.

8. **GMO Foods:**

- Genetically Modified Organisms: While controversial, some studies suggest that genetically modified foods may affect hormone balance and overall health, although more research is needed to fully understand their long-term effects.

Why Avoid These Foods?

- Disruption of Insulin and Leptin: Refined carbohydrates, sugars, and unhealthy fats can lead to insulin resistance and leptin resistance, disrupting appetite regulation, metabolism, and hormone balance.

- Inflammation: Many of these foods contribute to chronic inflammation, which interferes with hormone production, cellular communication, and overall health.

- Liver Overload: Alcohol and processed foods can strain the liver, reducing its ability to metabolize hormones and toxins effectively.

- Endocrine Disruption: Certain additives, chemicals, and

hormones in food products can mimic or interfere with natural hormone production and signaling pathways in the body. Avoiding these foods and making healthier choices can support hormone balance and overall well-being. It's essential to focus on a balanced diet rich in whole foods, lean proteins, healthy fats, and plenty of fruits and vegetables to promote optimal hormone function. Individual responses to these foods may vary, so it's beneficial to consult with a healthcare provider or registered dietitian to create a personalized nutrition plan that supports hormone balance based on individual health needs and goals.

Conclusion

To summarize, maintaining hormone balance through diet entails not only selecting helpful foods, but also avoiding or limiting items that can disrupt hormone production and overall health. Foods to avoid include refined carbs and sweets, trans fats, excessive coffee and alcohol, some soy products, conventional dairy (for some people), artificial sweeteners and additives, mercury-rich fish, and potentially GMO foods.

These meals can disrupt hormone homeostasis via a variety of processes. Refined carbs and sugars induce rapid spikes in blood sugar and insulin levels, resulting in insulin resistance and altering metabolic hormones such as insulin and leptin. Trans fats and harmful fats contribute to inflammation, which disrupts hormone production and function. Excessive caffeine and alcohol consumption can disturb cortisol levels, disrupt sleep patterns, and decreased adrenal function, all of which influence hormonal control. In sensitive individuals, compounds found in soy products and traditional dairy may mimic estrogen or interfere with hormone signaling. Artificial sweeteners, additives, and GMO foods may also be harmful to hormone health, but more research is needed to properly understand their effects.

Avoiding these foods promotes hormone balance by lowering inflammation, maintaining liver function (which is essential for hormone metabolism), and improving general metabolic health. Instead, a diet high in nutrient-dense whole foods, including lean proteins, healthy fats, colorful vegetables, fruits, whole grains, and herbs and spices, can supply critical nutrients and antioxidants that help with hormone synthesis, control, and overall well-being.

Individual reactions to various foods can differ, so it's critical to consider unique health conditions, sensitivities, and goals when making dietary decisions. Consulting with a healthcare professional or registered dietitian can provide tailored advice and assistance in developing a balanced nutrition plan that promotes optimal hormone balance and long-term health. Individuals who adopt a thoughtful approach to food choices and lifestyle behaviors can effectively boost their hormone health and improve their overall quality of life.